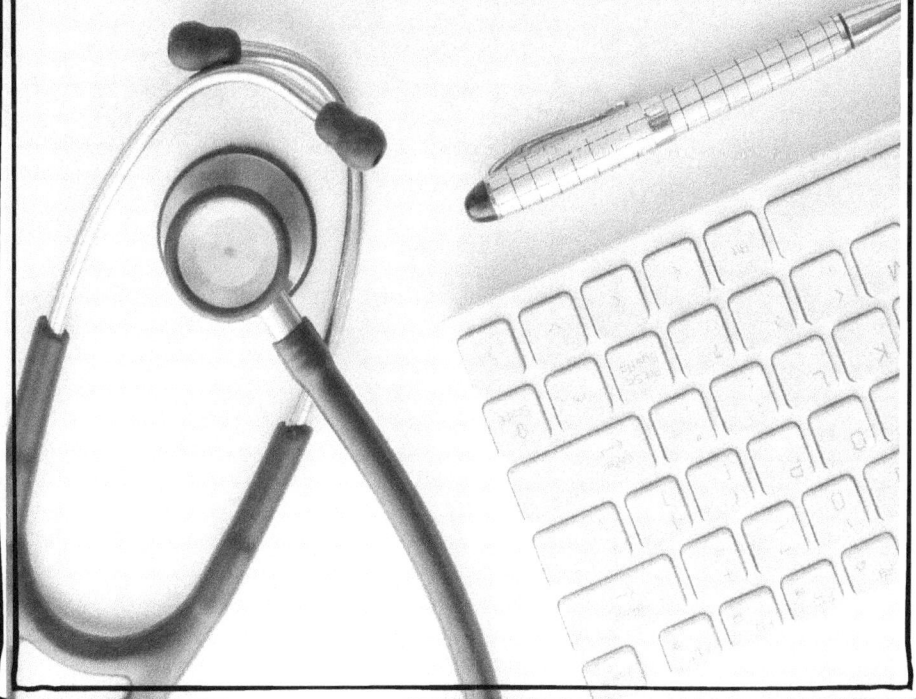

HOW TO BECOME A PROFESSIONAL DOCTOR

Copyright © 2024 by Preeti Rawat & B.S. Rawat

All rights reserved. No part of this book may be reproduced, distributed, or transmitted in any form or by any means, including photocopying, recording, or other electronic or mechanical methods, without the prior written permission of the author, except in the case of brief quotations embodied in critical reviews and certain other noncommercial uses permitted by copyright law.

Printed in India

First Edition: 2024

Disclaimer: The information contained in this book is for general informational purposes only. The author and publisher are not responsible for any errors or omissions, or for any consequences arising from the use of the information presented in this book.

Any resemblance to actual persons, living or dead, or actual events is purely coincidental.

Every effort has been made to ensure that the information in this book is accurate. However, the author and publisher do not assume any responsibility or liability for errors, inaccuracies, or omissions.

Preface

Welcome to "How to Become a Professional Doctor," a comprehensive guide designed to assist aspiring individuals in navigating the intricate journey towards a fulfilling career in medicine. As you hold this book in your hands, you may be filled with excitement, curiosity, or perhaps even a hint of apprehension about the path that lies ahead. Rest assured, you are not alone.

Embarking on the journey to become a doctor is akin to setting sail on a vast ocean, where the horizon stretches infinitely, and the destination may seem distant and uncertain. Yet, within these pages, you will find a detailed roadmap crafted to illuminate your path, guiding you through the ebbs and flows, the highs and lows, and the myriad choices that define this remarkable expedition.

Whether you are a high school student with dreams of healing, a college graduate contemplating a career change, or someone seeking to fulfill a lifelong ambition, this book is tailored to meet you where you are and empower you to chart your course towards becoming a professional doctor.

Within these chapters, you will discover insights garnered from seasoned professionals, practical advice distilled from years of experience, and actionable steps to propel you forward on your journey. From understanding the intricacies of medical education to navigating the complexities of residency training and beyond, each page is imbued with the wisdom and encouragement you need to thrive in the ever-evolving landscape of medicine.

As you embark on this odyssey, remember that the path to becoming a doctor is not merely a destination to reach but a transformative voyage to embrace fully. It is a journey of self-discovery, resilience, and unwavering dedication—a journey that will challenge you, shape you, and ultimately redefine you in profound ways.

So, with an open mind and a courageous heart, I invite you to embark on this adventure with me. Together, let us embark on a voyage of discovery, growth, and fulfillment—a journey that will not only lead us to the noble profession of medicine but also to a life of purpose, service, and meaning.

Bon voyage, dear reader, and may the pages that follow serve as your steadfast companion on the extraordinary voyage to becoming a professional doctor.

Warm regards,

Preeti Rawat

B.S. Rawat

Content

S.No.	Chapters
1	Understanding the Path to Medicine
2	Preparing for Medical School
3	Excelling in Medical School
4	Choosing a Speciality
5	Residency and Fellowship Training
6	Transitioning to Practice
7	Thriving as a Professional Doctor

Introduction

Becoming a professional doctor is a journey filled with challenges, sacrifices, and countless hours of dedication. However, it is also one of the most rewarding and fulfilling careers one can pursue. This book is your comprehensive guide to navigating this journey, from choosing the right educational path to excelling in your practice. Whether you're a high school student dreaming of a career in medicine or a professional considering a career change, this book will provide you with the essential knowledge and strategies to succeed in becoming a doctor.

Chapter 1: Understanding the Path to Medicine

- Exploring the different fields of medicine

- Understanding the educational requirements

- Evaluating personal motivations and goals

Chapter 2: Preparing for Medical School

- Building a strong academic foundation

- Gaining relevant volunteer and work experience

- Navigating the medical school application process

Chapter 3: Excelling in Medical School

- Mastering effective study techniques

- Balancing academic demands with personal well-being

- Building strong relationships with peers and mentors

Chapter 4: Choosing a Specialty

- Exploring various medical specialties

- Assessing personal interests, strengths, and values

- Gaining exposure through clinical rotations and electives

Chapter 5: Residency and Fellowship Training

- Understanding the residency match process

- Excelling during residency and fellowship training

- Building a strong professional network

Chapter 6: Transitioning to Practice

- Navigating the job search process

- Understanding the business side of medicine

- Cultivating effective communication and patient care skills

Chapter 7: Thriving as a Professional Doctor

- Maintaining work-life balance

- Continuing professional development

- Navigating challenges and obstacles

Chapter 1

Understanding the Path to Medicine

Embarking on the journey to become a doctor is a significant decision that requires careful consideration and a deep understanding of the path ahead. In this chapter, we will explore the multifaceted nature of the medical profession, from the diverse fields of practice to the educational requirements and personal motivations that drive individuals to pursue this noble career.

1.1 Exploring the Different Fields of Medicine

Medicine encompasses a vast array of specialties and subspecialties, each offering unique opportunities for professional growth and fulfillment. From primary care specialties such as family medicine, internal medicine, and pediatrics to surgical disciplines like orthopedic surgery, neurosurgery, and cardiothoracic surgery, the options are as diverse as the patients they serve.

As you begin your journey, take the time to explore the various fields of medicine and consider which aligns most closely with your interests, values, and long-term career goals. Engage in shadowing experiences, volunteer work, and informational interviews to gain insight into the day-to-day responsibilities, challenges, and rewards associated with different specialties.

1.2 Understanding the Educational Requirements

Becoming a doctor requires a rigorous educational journey that typically begins with earning a bachelor's degree followed by completion of medical school and residency training. The specific requirements may vary depending on the country and region in which you intend to practice, so it is essential to research and understand the educational pathways available to you.

In most cases, admission to medical school is highly competitive and requires a strong academic record, satisfactory performance on standardized tests such as the MCAT (Medical College Admission Test), and compelling personal statements and letters of recommendation. Once accepted, medical school typically consists of four years of intensive coursework, clinical rotations, and examinations culminating in the awarding of a Doctor of Medicine (MD) or Doctor of Osteopathic Medicine (DO) degree.

Following medical school, aspiring doctors must complete residency training in their chosen specialty, which can range from three to seven years or more depending on the field. Residency provides hands-on clinical experience under the supervision of experienced physicians and is a critical step in preparing for independent practice.

1.3 Evaluating Personal Motivations and Goals

Beyond academic achievements and clinical skills, a career in medicine requires a deep-seated commitment to serving others and a genuine passion for healing. Take the time to reflect on your personal motivations for pursuing a career in medicine and consider how your values, experiences, and aspirations align with the demands of the profession.

Ask yourself what drives you to become a doctor and what impact you hope to make in the lives of your patients and communities. Whether it is a desire to alleviate suffering, promote health equity, or advance medical knowledge through research, understanding your underlying motivations will sustain you through the challenges and uncertainties that lie ahead.

In conclusion, understanding the path to medicine is the first step in embarking on this transformative journey. By exploring the diverse fields of medicine, understanding the educational requirements, and evaluating your personal motivations and goals, you will lay a solid foundation for success as you pursue your dreams of becoming a professional doctor.

Chapter 2

Preparing for Medical School

Preparing for medical school is a crucial phase in the journey to becoming a doctor. It requires diligent planning, dedicated effort, and a commitment to academic excellence. In this chapter, we will explore the essential steps you can take to strengthen your candidacy, maximize your chances of admission, and lay the groundwork for success in medical school.

2.1 Building a Strong Academic Foundation

Academic excellence is a cornerstone of medical school admissions. Medical schools typically seek candidates with strong undergraduate records, particularly in science-related coursework. As you progress through your undergraduate studies, prioritize your academic performance by:

- Taking challenging coursework in biology, chemistry, physics, and mathematics to build a solid foundation in the sciences.

- Maintaining a competitive GPA (Grade Point Average) by staying organized, managing your time effectively, and seeking academic support when needed.

- Demonstrating your intellectual curiosity and passion for learning through participation in research projects, honors programs, and advanced coursework.

Remember that academic achievement is not solely measured by grades; admissions committees also value qualities such as critical thinking, problem-solving skills, and intellectual curiosity.

2.2 Gaining Relevant Volunteer and Work Experience

In addition to academic excellence, medical schools value candidates who demonstrate a commitment to service and a genuine interest in healthcare. Seek out opportunities to gain firsthand experience in clinical settings, volunteer organizations, and healthcare-related roles, such as:

- Volunteering at hospitals, clinics, or community health centers to gain exposure to patient care and healthcare delivery.

- Shadowing physicians in various specialties to observe clinical practice and gain insight into the daily responsibilities of a doctor.

- Participating in medical mission trips, community outreach programs, or health education initiatives to make a meaningful impact in underserved communities.

These experiences not only enrich your understanding of medicine but also demonstrate your compassion, empathy, and commitment to serving others—qualities that are highly valued by medical school admissions committees.

2.3 Navigating the Medical School Application Process

The medical school application process can be daunting, but with careful preparation and attention to detail, you can present yourself as a competitive candidate. Here are key steps to navigate the application process successfully:

- Research medical schools thoroughly to identify programs that align with your interests, values, and career goals.

- Prepare for and take the MCAT (Medical College Admission Test) or other required standardized tests, dedicating ample time to study and practice.

- Craft a compelling personal statement that highlights your motivations for pursuing a career in medicine, relevant experiences, and personal qualities.

- Secure strong letters of recommendation from professors, mentors, or healthcare professionals who can attest to your academic abilities, character, and suitability for medical school.

- Complete the application materials accurately and submit them by the specified deadlines, paying close attention to each school's requirements and preferences.

By approaching the application process strategically and presenting a well-rounded portfolio of academic achievements, extracurricular activities, and personal qualities, you can enhance your chances of securing admission to medical school.

In conclusion, preparing for medical school requires a holistic approach that encompasses academic excellence, relevant experiences, and careful attention to the application process. By building a strong academic foundation, gaining meaningful volunteer and work experience, and navigating the application process with diligence and purpose, you can position yourself for success as you embark on the next phase of your journey to becoming a professional doctor.

Chapter 3

Excelling in Medical School

Entering medical school marks the beginning of a transformative journey that will shape you intellectually, professionally, and personally.

Excelling in medical school requires more than just academic prowess; it demands resilience, adaptability, and a commitment to lifelong learning. In this chapter, we will explore the essential strategies and skills you need to thrive in medical school and lay the foundation for a successful career in medicine.

3.1 Mastering Effective Study Techniques

Medical school curriculum is rigorous and demanding, encompassing a vast array of scientific principles, clinical skills, and medical knowledge. To succeed academically, it is essential to develop effective study techniques that maximize your learning and retention. Consider implementing the following strategies:

- Utilize active learning methods such as concept mapping, problem-based learning, and group discussions to engage with the material actively and deepen your understanding.

- Create a structured study schedule that allocates dedicated time for coursework, review sessions, and self-assessment.

- Employ spaced repetition techniques to reinforce learning over time and prevent forgetting.

- Seek out resources such as textbooks, online modules, and educational videos to supplement your coursework and enhance your understanding of challenging concepts.

By adopting a proactive approach to studying and experimenting with different techniques, you can optimize your learning experience and excel academically in medical school.

3.2 Balancing Academic Demands with Personal Well-being

Medical school can be intense and demanding, often requiring long hours of study, clinical rotations, and extracurricular activities.

However, it is essential to prioritize your physical, mental, and emotional well-being to maintain a healthy balance and prevent burnout. Consider the following strategies for self-care:

- Prioritize adequate sleep, nutrition, and exercise to support your physical health and cognitive function.

- Practice stress management techniques such as mindfulness meditation, deep breathing exercises, and progressive muscle relaxation to reduce anxiety and promote relaxation.

- Cultivate a supportive network of friends, family members, peers, and mentors who can offer encouragement, advice, and emotional support.

- Set realistic goals and expectations for yourself, recognizing that perfection is unattainable and that it is okay to ask for help when needed.

Remember that self-care is not a luxury but a necessity for long-term success and well-being in medical school and beyond.

3.3 Building Strong Relationships with Peers and Mentors

Medical school is as much about collaboration and teamwork as it is about individual achievement. Cultivating strong relationships with your peers and mentors can enhance your learning experience, provide valuable support, and foster personal growth. Consider the following strategies for building meaningful connections:

- Actively participate in group study sessions, student organizations, and extracurricular activities to connect with your classmates and engage in collaborative learning.

- Seek out mentors—faculty members, senior students, or practicing physicians—who can offer guidance, advice, and career support.

- Embrace diversity and inclusivity by engaging with individuals from different backgrounds, cultures, and perspectives.

- Pay it forward by supporting and mentoring junior students, sharing your knowledge and experiences, and contributing to a culture of collaboration and mutual respect.

By investing in relationships with your peers and mentors, you can create a supportive community that enriches your medical school experience and lays the groundwork for professional success.

In conclusion, excelling in medical school requires more than just academic aptitude; it demands resilience, self-care, and meaningful connections with peers and mentors. By mastering effective study techniques, prioritizing your well-being, and building strong relationships, you can navigate the challenges of medical school with confidence and lay the foundation for a successful career in medicine.

Chapter 4

Choosing a Specialty

Choosing a medical specialty is a significant decision that will shape the trajectory of your career and professional identity. With a multitude of specialties and subspecialties available, each offering unique opportunities and challenges, it is essential to approach this decision thoughtfully and intentionally. In this chapter, we will explore the factors to consider when choosing a specialty, the process of exploration and decision-making, and strategies for gaining exposure to different fields of medicine.

4.1 Exploring Various Medical Specialties

The field of medicine is incredibly diverse, encompassing a wide range of specialties and subspecialties, each with its own focus, patient population, and clinical practice. From primary care disciplines such as family medicine, internal medicine, and pediatrics to surgical specialties like orthopedic surgery, neurosurgery, and cardiothoracic surgery, the options are vast and varied.

Take the time to explore the different medical specialties through:

- Clinical rotations: Participate in clinical rotations during medical school to gain exposure to various specialties and subspecialties. Pay attention to the types of patients you enjoy working with, the procedures that interest you, and the clinical environments where you feel most comfortable.

- Specialty electives: Take advantage of elective opportunities to delve deeper into specific areas of interest and gain hands-on experience under the guidance of experienced physicians.

- Shadowing experiences: Shadow physicians in different specialties to observe their day-to-day responsibilities, patient interactions, and clinical decision-making processes.

- Informational interviews: Speak with practicing physicians in various specialties to learn more about their career paths, professional satisfaction, and the pros and cons of their chosen specialties.

By exploring the diverse landscape of medical specialties, you can gain insight into the options available to you and begin to narrow down your areas of interest.

4.2 Assessing Personal Interests, Strengths, and Values

As you explore different medical specialties, it is essential to reflect on your personal interests, strengths, and values to identify the specialty that aligns most closely with your goals and aspirations. Consider the following questions:

- What aspects of medicine do you find most fulfilling and rewarding?

- What patient populations do you feel drawn to serving?

- What clinical environments and practice settings do you envision yourself thriving in?

- What procedural skills and clinical competencies are you most interested in developing?

- What lifestyle considerations and work-life balance are important to you?

By aligning your career choices with your personal interests, strengths, and values, you can ensure a more fulfilling and sustainable career in medicine.

4.3 Gaining Exposure through Clinical Rotations and Electives

Clinical rotations and elective experiences offer invaluable opportunities to gain hands-on experience in different medical specialties, interact with patients and healthcare teams, and refine your clinical skills and decision-making abilities. Be proactive in seeking out diverse clinical experiences and consider the following strategies:

- Rotate through a variety of clinical settings, including inpatient wards, outpatient clinics, emergency departments, and specialty clinics, to gain exposure to different patient populations and practice environments.

- Seek out elective opportunities in specialties that interest you, even if they are not required for your core curriculum. Use these experiences to explore your interests further and gain insight into the day-to-day realities of different specialties.

- Request feedback from supervising physicians, nurses, and other healthcare professionals to identify your strengths, areas for improvement, and potential fit with different specialties.

By actively engaging in clinical rotations and elective experiences, you can gain firsthand exposure to different medical specialties, clarify your career goals, and make informed decisions about your future specialty choice.

In conclusion, choosing a medical specialty is a significant decision that requires careful consideration of your interests, strengths, and values. By exploring various medical specialties, assessing your personal preferences, and gaining exposure through clinical rotations and electives, you can identify the specialty that aligns best with your career goals and embark on a rewarding and fulfilling career path in medicine.

Chapter 5

Residency and Fellowship Training

Entering residency and fellowship training marks a pivotal phase in your journey to becoming a fully-fledged physician. These postgraduate training programs provide the opportunity to develop clinical expertise, refine procedural skills, and gain practical experience under the supervision of experienced mentors. In this chapter, we will explore the residency match process, the structure of residency and fellowship training, and strategies for excelling in these programs.

5.1 Understanding the Residency Match Process

The residency match process, administered by organizations such as the National Resident Matching Program (NRMP) in the United States, is a highly competitive and structured system for allocating residency positions to medical graduates. Key elements of the match process include:

- Application: Submitting applications through centralized platforms such as the Electronic Residency Application Service (ERAS) and completing interviews with residency programs.

- Rank Order List: Ranking residency programs in order of preference based on factors such as program reputation, location, and specialty-specific attributes.

- Match Day: Receiving notification of residency program placement through the NRMP match algorithm and officially committing to the matched program.

Navigating the residency match process requires careful planning, preparation, and strategic decision-making to maximize your chances of securing a residency position in your desired specialty and location.

5.2 Excelling During Residency Training

Residency training is a rigorous and immersive experience that combines clinical rotations, didactic education, and hands-on patient care responsibilities. Key components of residency training include:

- Clinical Rotations: Rotating through various specialties and subspecialties to gain exposure to different patient populations, clinical settings, and disease processes.

- Supervised Patient Care: Providing direct patient care under the supervision of attending physicians, residents, and interdisciplinary healthcare teams.

- Didactic Education: Participating in lectures, seminars, grand rounds, and case conferences to expand your medical knowledge and enhance your clinical reasoning skills.

- Professional Development: Engaging in scholarly activities, quality improvement projects, and research endeavors to contribute to the advancement of medical knowledge and practice.

To excel during residency training, it is essential to demonstrate clinical competence, professionalism, and a commitment to lifelong learning. Seek out opportunities for mentorship, feedback, and self-reflection to maximize your growth and development as a physician.

5.3 Pursuing Fellowship Training

For some medical specialties, fellowship training offers advanced subspecialty training and specialization beyond residency. Fellowship programs provide the opportunity to deepen your expertise in a specific area of medicine, conduct research, and become a leader in your field. Key considerations when pursuing fellowship training include:

- Identifying Career Goals: Clarify your career objectives and assess whether fellowship training aligns with your long-term professional aspirations.

- Researching Fellowship Programs: Research fellowship programs thoroughly to identify those that offer comprehensive training, mentorship opportunities, and a supportive learning environment.

- Application and Match Process: Navigate the fellowship match process, which may involve submitting applications through centralized platforms such as ERAS and participating in interviews with fellowship programs.

By pursuing fellowship training, you can enhance your clinical skills, broaden your career opportunities, and make a meaningful contribution to your chosen field of medicine.

In conclusion, residency and fellowship training are integral components of the journey to becoming a proficient physician. By understanding the residency match process, excelling during residency training, and pursuing fellowship opportunities strategically, you can lay the groundwork for a successful and fulfilling career in medicine.

Chapter 6

Transitioning to Practice

Transitioning from residency or fellowship training to independent practice marks a significant milestone in your career as a physician. As you embark on this journey, you will encounter new challenges, responsibilities, and opportunities for professional growth. In this chapter, we will explore the key considerations and strategies for navigating the transition to practice successfully.

6.1 Navigating the Job Search Process

The job search process can be overwhelming, but with careful planning and preparation, you can find opportunities that align with your career goals and aspirations. Consider the following steps when navigating the job search process:

- Define Your Priorities: Clarify your preferences regarding practice setting, geographic location, patient population, and work-life balance to narrow down your job search criteria.

- Research Opportunities: Explore job openings through online job boards, professional networking platforms, and specialty-specific organizations. Consider reaching out to colleagues, mentors, and alumni for recommendations and referrals.

- Tailor Your Application Materials: Customize your curriculum vitae (CV), cover letter, and other application materials to highlight your relevant experience, skills, and accomplishments. Emphasize how your background aligns with the specific requirements and priorities of each position.

- Prepare for Interviews: Prepare thoroughly for interviews by researching prospective employers, practicing common interview questions, and articulating your career goals and strengths effectively. Consider seeking feedback from mentors or colleagues to enhance your interview performance.

- Negotiate Compensation and Benefits: Evaluate job offers carefully, considering factors such as salary, benefits, professional development opportunities, and contract terms. Negotiate effectively to ensure that the terms of employment are fair and equitable.

By approaching the job search process strategically and thoughtfully, you can identify opportunities that match your professional goals and preferences.

6.2 Understanding the Business Side of Medicine

Transitioning to independent practice requires a solid understanding of the business aspects of medicine, including practice management, billing and coding, and compliance regulations. Consider the following considerations when navigating the business side of medicine:

- Practice Management: Familiarize yourself with the operational aspects of running a medical practice, including staffing, scheduling, workflow optimization, and patient engagement strategies.

- Billing and Coding: Learn the fundamentals of medical billing and coding to ensure accurate and timely reimbursement for the services you provide. Stay informed about changes to coding guidelines, documentation requirements, and payer policies to avoid billing errors and compliance issues.

- Compliance Regulations: Stay abreast of healthcare laws, regulations, and standards of practice to ensure compliance with legal and ethical guidelines. Familiarize yourself with

HIPAA (Health Insurance Portability and Accountability Act) regulations, Stark Law, anti-kickback statutes, and other relevant laws that govern the practice of medicine.

By acquiring knowledge and skills in practice management, billing and coding, and compliance regulations, you can navigate the business side of medicine with confidence and integrity.

6.3 Cultivating Effective Communication and Patient Care Skills

Effective communication and patient care skills are essential for building trust, fostering therapeutic relationships, and delivering high-quality care to patients. Consider the following strategies for cultivating these skills:

- Active Listening: Practice active listening by giving patients your full attention, asking open-ended questions, and validating their concerns and perspectives. Demonstrate empathy, compassion, and respect in your interactions with patients and their families.

- Clear and Concise Communication: Communicate medical information in clear, understandable language, avoiding jargon and technical terminology. Use visual aids, diagrams, and illustrations as needed to enhance patient understanding.

- Cultural Competence: Respect and honor the cultural backgrounds, beliefs, and values of your patients. Recognize the impact of cultural factors on health beliefs, treatment preferences, and healthcare decision-making.

- Interdisciplinary Collaboration: Collaborate effectively with other healthcare professionals, including nurses, pharmacists, social workers, and allied health professionals, to coordinate care and optimize patient outcomes. Value the expertise and contributions of each team member and foster a culture of mutual respect and collaboration.

By prioritizing effective communication and patient-centered care, you can enhance the quality of care you provide and strengthen the patient-provider relationship.

In conclusion, transitioning to independent practice requires careful planning, preparation, and ongoing professional development. By navigating the job search process strategically, understanding the business side of medicine, and cultivating effective communication and patient care skills, you can embark on a successful and fulfilling career as a practicing physician.

Chapter 7
Thriving as a Professional Doctor

Thriving as a professional doctor goes beyond clinical competence; it encompasses personal fulfillment, professional growth, and a commitment to lifelong learning and well-being. In this chapter, we will explore strategies for maintaining work-life balance, continuing professional development, and navigating the challenges and opportunities of the medical profession.

7.1 Maintaining Work-Life Balance

Work-life balance is essential for sustaining long-term well-being and preventing burnout in the demanding field of medicine. Consider the following strategies for achieving and maintaining balance in your personal and professional life:

- Set Boundaries: Establish clear boundaries between work and personal life by defining dedicated time for rest, relaxation, and leisure activities. Prioritize activities that bring you joy and fulfillment outside of medicine.

- Practice Self-Care: Prioritize self-care practices such as exercise, mindfulness meditation, hobbies, and social connections to recharge and rejuvenate your mind, body, and spirit.

- Delegate Responsibilities: Delegate tasks and responsibilities whenever possible to lighten your workload and create space for self-care and personal pursuits. Collaborate with colleagues, support staff, and interdisciplinary teams to share the workload effectively.

- Seek Support: Reach out to colleagues, mentors, friends, and family members for support, encouragement, and perspective during challenging times. Consider joining peer support groups, counseling services, or wellness initiatives to connect with others who share similar experiences and concerns.

By prioritizing work-life balance and self-care, you can enhance your resilience, prevent burnout, and sustain a fulfilling and sustainable career in medicine.

7.2 Continuing Professional Development

Continuing professional development is essential for staying current with advances in medical knowledge, technology, and practice standards. Consider the following strategies for lifelong learning and professional growth:

- Engage in Continuing Education: Participate in conferences, workshops, seminars, and online courses to expand your medical knowledge, enhance your clinical skills, and stay abreast of emerging trends and best practices in your specialty.

- Pursue Board Certification: Consider pursuing board certification in your specialty or subspecialty to demonstrate your expertise, commitment to excellence, and dedication to ongoing professional development. Maintain certification through regular participation in continuing medical education (CME) activities and recertification exams as required.

- Participate in Research and Scholarship: Engage in scholarly activities such as research projects, quality improvement initiatives, and clinical trials to contribute to the advancement of medical knowledge and practice. Collaborate with colleagues, mentor junior trainees, and publish your findings in peer-reviewed journals to disseminate knowledge and innovation within the medical community.

- Mentorship and Teaching: Serve as a mentor and educator for medical students, residents, and junior colleagues to share your knowledge, skills, and expertise. Foster a culture of learning and professional development within your institution by providing guidance, feedback, and support to aspiring healthcare professionals.

By embracing lifelong learning and professional development, you can enhance your clinical expertise, advance your career, and make a meaningful contribution to the field of medicine.

7.3 Navigating Challenges and Opportunities

The medical profession is dynamic and ever-evolving, presenting both challenges and opportunities for growth and adaptation. Consider the following strategies for navigating the complexities of the medical landscape:

- Embrace Change: Embrace change as an opportunity for growth and innovation, rather than a source of fear or resistance. Stay flexible, open-minded, and adaptable in the face of evolving practice standards, technologies, and healthcare delivery models.

- Advocate for Patients and Profession: Advocate for the needs and interests of your patients, colleagues, and profession by actively participating in professional organizations, policy initiatives, and public health campaigns. Champion initiatives that promote patient safety, access to care, and healthcare equity within your community and beyond.

- Cultivate Resilience: Cultivate resilience by developing coping strategies, positive mindset, and social support networks to navigate challenges, setbacks, and adversity with grace and perseverance. Draw upon your inner strengths, values, and sense of purpose to overcome obstacles and thrive in the face of adversity.

- Foster Collegiality and Collaboration: Foster a culture of collegiality, collaboration, and mutual respect within your workplace and professional community. Build strong relationships with colleagues, support staff, and interdisciplinary teams based on trust, communication, and shared goals.

By embracing challenges as opportunities for growth, advocating for your patients and profession, cultivating resilience, and fostering collaboration, you can navigate the complexities of the medical profession with confidence and integrity.

In conclusion, thriving as a professional doctor requires a holistic approach that encompasses work-life balance, continuing professional development, and resilience in the face of challenges and opportunities. By prioritizing self-care, lifelong learning, and advocacy, you can sustain a fulfilling and impactful career in medicine while making a meaningful difference in the lives of others.

About The Author

Dear Reader,

As you journey through the pages of **"How to Become a Professional Doctor,"** I extend my warmest congratulations on taking the first steps towards a career in medicine. Whether you're a student exploring your options, a recent graduate navigating the residency match process, or a seasoned physician seeking guidance on professional development, I wrote this book with you in mind.

In writing this book, my goal is to provide you with a roadmap—a guiding light to navigate the complexities of medical education, residency training, and professional practice. Drawing upon my own experiences, as well as the wisdom of mentors, colleagues, and peers, I have distilled practical advice, actionable strategies, and heartfelt encouragement to support you on your journey.

I believe that becoming a professional doctor is not just about acquiring knowledge and skills; it is a transformative journey of self-discovery, growth, and service to others. It is a calling—a privilege and a responsibility—to heal, comfort, and advocate for those in need. As you embark on this journey, I invite you to embrace the challenges, cherish the triumphs, and never lose sight of the profound impact you can make in the lives of your patients and communities.

May this book serve as a trusted companion, offering guidance, inspiration, and reassurance as you navigate the path to becoming a professional doctor. Remember, you are not alone. Together, let us honor the legacy of those who came before us and inspire the generations that follow to uphold the highest ideals of medicine.

With heartfelt wishes for your success and fulfillment,

Preeti Rawat

B.S. Rawat

www.ingramcontent.com/pod-product-compliance
Lightning Source LLC
Chambersburg PA
CBHW070416230526
45471CB00006B/2828